THE KEY TO GOOD

HEALTH AND LONGEVITY:

BCOME YOUR FIRST DOCTOR

AND

LIVE HEALTHY

LIFE

ANGELO O. ONEKA

TABLE OF CONTENTS

CHAPTER

PREFACE

We all long for good health, because when we have good health, we are not only happy, but are

also able to work and bring improvements in our lives.

Good health can also lead us to longevity. And there can never be longevity without good health.

To achieve good health, we need to practise the discipline of hygiene and other related health

disciplines. And if we routinely practise the requirements of good health, then good health becomes

achievable. Alternatively, if we ignore and neglect these requirements, that means we are heading

for poor health. And poor health can not only be a nuisance but can also deprive us the happiness in

life. It may also impose on us poverty, which will yet cause us more problems.

As the title of the book indicates, we can greatly improve our health by becoming our first doctors.

This can not only bring improvements in our health but it will also protect us from being easily

vunerable to diseases. Remember, before medical schools, there were doctors, and before medical doctors, there were doctors.

Treatments were being administered by people who never went to medical schools, and there were successful treatments as well as failures, just as they are also today. And therefore, by becoming your first doctor, you are not only paving your way to good health and happiness, but you are also paving your way to longevity.

This book is written to show you many of the things we take for guaranted that can greatly improve our health and also protect us from diseases and things that could harm us and deny us good health and happiness. It will also show you things that you need to avoid in order to be healthy and avoid premature death.

CHAPTER 1   PERSONAL HYGIENE

Personal hygiene is very important in keeping with good health. If you want to have good health and

avoid frequently becoming sick, then you critically need to observe personal hygiene. People who do

not observe personal hygiene, frequently fall sick.

Personal hygiene may include the following:

1. Taking care of your nails

2. Washing your hands regularly

3. Taking care of your teeth

4. Taking care of your hair

5. Having shower or taking bath regularly

6. Taking care of your ears

7. Taking care of your nose

TAKING CARE OF YOUR NAILS

Taking care of your nails is very important for your good health. We need to take care of our nails for

a number of reasons. One of them is to look clean and smart. People may judge whether a person is

a clean or dirty person by simply looking at his or her nails. Dirty nails indicate that a person is a dirty

person, especially if the nails are not cut short and look dirty.

The most important reason, however, is hygiene. Since we use our hands for various purposes, such

as doing the work, lifting things, as well as for eating, we have therefore ought to be very careful and

to make sure that our nails are kept short and clean, especially when it comes to eating.

Sickness and even death may occur when after doing a dirty work or handling something poisonous

and we eat without thoroughly washing our nails, especially under them. As we lick our fingers in the

process of eating, we may be swallowing dirt or even poison into our stomachs. And that will cause

us to become sick or even die. These are not all the long and dirty nails may cause us.

By having long and dirty nails, we may also accidentally scratch injure ourselves. And if the caused wounds become infected because of poor hygiene that we may be accustomed to, it may lead to serious problems.

Also they may accidentally injure other people, say in a play, or in a crowded place when you may be adjusting the position of your hand. Or when you are taking care of a baby, you may also accidentally injure that baby. The list may go on and on.

WASH YOUR HANDS REGULARLY

The washing of hands on a regular basis is a preventive measure. Our hands are good servants that do most of the work without complaints.

We use our hands to do various activities; to do work, to lift things, to write, to shake fellow hands, to eat, etc. Life and death are also in the hands. When we work, the hands are virtually giving us life and when we eat with hands that are fully contaminated with dangerous chemicals or poison, it is death in the lurking.

Because of the fear of sickness and death that is why we should always wash our hands before eating even if you may be using cutleries, for you never know when you are going to touch the food you are eating. Unclean hand has a lot of dangers.

THE DANGERS OF NOT WASHING THE HANDS

There can be a lot of serious dangers if we do not wash our hands regularly. Some of these dangers

are:

1. You could easily poison yourself.

2. You could cause yourself to become blind.

3. You could infect your private part.

4. You could easily poison others.

5. You could transmit germs to other people.

6. You could contaminate appliances and other tools, etc.

7. If you have flu, you could infect other people.

YOU COULD EASILY POISON YOURSELF

If you do not wash your hands after work, lifting something or touching something dirty or

contaminated, and you use those hands to eat, you could end up poisoning yourself. And this

may lead to serious consequences, including death.

It is therefore important that after every work you do, lifting up things or touching anything

dirty, you should always wash your hands for preventive purposes. As the saying goes '

prevention is better than cure'.

YOU COULD CAUSE YOURSELF TO BECOME BLIND

Also if you do not wash your hands after work, lifting something or touching something dirty,

you could easily cause yourself to become blind, especially if you happen to rub your eyes

with those contaminated hands.

YOU COULD INFECT YOUR PRIVATE PART

In the same manner, if you do not wash your hands after work, lifting something dirty or touching something contaminated, and you touch your private part with those contaminated hands, you could easily infect it, and this may lead to serious problems.

YOU COULD EASILY POISON OTHERS

As you could poison yourself, you could also poison other people that you great with your dirty hands, if they fall in your category of not washing their hands before eating.

YOU COULD TRANSMIT GERMS TO OTHER PEOPLE

If you had been working in a germ infested area and you happen to shake hands with other people before washing your hands, you could easily transmit the germs to those people.

YOU COULD CONTAMINATE APPLIANCES AND OTHER THINGS YOU TOUCH

Again, if you were working in a dirty or contaminated place, and you come home, open the fridge, operate the TV or music system, touch remote controls, etc., without first washing your hands, you could easily contaminate those things and seriously cause serious problems to others as well as yourself.

IF YOU HAVE THE FLU, YOU COULD EASILY TRANSMIT IT TO OTHERS

Hhappen to be one of them and you happen to have colds, and also happen to shake the hands of other people, you could easily transmit the virus to them.

THE DANGERS OF HANDSHAKE

Handshake can be quite a dangerous hidden destruction. There are many reasons why it may be very fatal. One of them is that many people do not care to wash their hands after handling dangerous substances or after using the washrooms. And when you shake their dirty hands, they are virtually transferring those dangerous substances or the germs into your hand. Others blow their noses with their naked hands and thereafter rub the mucus into their hands, such hands are seriously contaminated and a handshake means getting the virus or the germs from them.

It is therefore advisable to wash your hands at regular intervals or whenever you are going to eat anything. Do not take anything for guaranted, as doing so would risk your health.

SANITIZER

Sanitizer is effective for killing germs but do not use it in lieu of water to clean your hands when you are going to eat. If you use sanitizer as a means to clean your hands whenever you are going to eat, you will simply be poisoning yourself, especially when you lick your fingers. Play safe and always wash your hands before eating.

TAKING CARE OF YOUR TEETH

If you always take care of your teeth, then you have no need for the dentists.

To avoid suffering from terrible pains that decayed teeth will give you, always brush your teeth every morning and every night before going to bed. If possible also brush your teeth after every meal. This will clear the food from your teeth, however, if you leave the food on your teeth, it can easily cause them to decay.

Floshing is also very important to keep the teeth clean and avoid tooth decay. If you do not flosh your teeth often, you can have smelling mouth that smells like the sewage because of the food that is stuck between your teeth. Floshing is another preventive measure to avoid tooth-decay.

TAKING CARE OF YOUR HAIR

You hair talks a lot about you. Poorly groomed hair tells people you have some kind of problems and smartly groomed hair tells people that you are okay and possibly successful. Have you ever seen any President, Prime Minister, a King, a Chief, etc., come out with ungroomed hair? They come out with well -groomed hair. A complete reflection of their status and success.

I love grooming my hair. I have been doing this since childhood. Now I have even less work to do to my head because of the airfield in my head.

Besides those indicated reasons, ungroomed hair gives people a conclusion that you are probably, a lazy and a dirty person. And groomed hair would say the opposite, that you are a clean person.

Again, if you do not properly groom your hair, the lice might inhabit there, and that is not only shameful but also a nuisance.

Besides lice, you could also have dandruffs. This is yet another nuisance of not properly taking care of your hair.

Yet still, people may mistake you for a mad person. You may also be ostracized because of your appearance, and it is equally possible that you may lose friends.

Yet another problem that might surface, is that as you have the lice, you may also end up having scabies.

THE EARS

The ears are among the very important parts of our bodies. The ears have a lot of functions for your wellbeing. Some of these functions are:

Hearing. Obviously, hearing comes first and foremost.

The ears as the eyes, are protective parts of our bodies. The alert us of any danger that might be brewing up, e.g., if you are crossing the road or rail line, they will alert you of the approaching vehicles or a train.

In a dangerous war zone, they alert you of the approaching enemies by the sounds of gun fires. Where construction work is taking place, they warn you of the falling dangerous debris. And when people are plotting to harm or kill you, when you hear of the plot, you will escape or take maximum precaution.

The ears also can entertain you, for example, one is only able to enjoy the music when the ears receive it and transmit it to the brain and body. Besides all these, the ears are very important means of receiving education. In the classrooms, you attentively listen to the teachers who are imparting into the knowledge.

Being important part of our bodies, we therefore have to make sure that we take care of them. And how do we take care of our ears? We can take care of our ears in many ways. Some of these ways are:

a. Regularly, we have to remove the pilling wax from our ears, that we may be able, to hear well.

b. In a noisy place, such as the factories, we can protect our ears by wearing earplugs.

c. We also have to make sure that dangerous things, such as dangerous chemicals, do not enter into our ears, by staying away from such places that contain them, or by wearing earplugs.

d. We should avoid putting dirty things, fingers, or sharp things into our ears, whenever they are hitching.

e. We should also avoid putting things we are not sure of, into our ears.

And foremost, if you have any problem with your ears, you should waste no time but see the ear specialist in order to diagnose the problem and receive a proper treatment accordingly. However, if you delay in seeing the doctor, this simple problem, may turn into major problem, and you may even lose your hearing.

Can you imagine what life will be like when you happen to lose your hearing! That spells a lot of problems. It may also require you to undergo special training to be able to associate and communicate with other people. Another alternative would possibly be to acquire a hearing device.

THE NOSE

The nose is another important part of the body. The nose plays very essential function to the body. The very essential function is to smell. It smells both the good and the bad, the dangerous as well as the non-dangerous smells and transmits these to the brain who then analyses and transmits to the whole body.

Following the brain transmission to the whole body, the reaction then sets in. If it is a dangerous thing, then the body is automatically affected, hence with serious consequences. And if it is a non-dangerous thing and it is something good and inviting, the body is thus stimulated to this. If it is the smell of something edible, the appetite is thus fully aroused. Sometimes as a result, we begin to feel hungry too.

What we smell can whet our appetite or spells illness or even death itself. Sometimes even the smell of something edible may spell illness or even death for us, especially when we have allergy problems. Just like in the case of peanuts or peanut butter, people who are allergic to them, have serious problem whenever they come into contact with the smell.

The nose therefore, seems to play the role of a whistle blower. It warns us to stay away from things that may be dangerous to our bodies. Alternatively, it also acts the role of invitation. It tells us something good and edible is here, come partake of it.

When something is good and helpful to you, you should always protect it. And how do we render back to the nose? There are many measures we can undertake to safeguard our noses. Some of these are:

DO NOT POKE YOUR NOSE

Nose poking can at times turns out to be very dangerous, especially if one had been handling something dangerous. If you had been handling something dangerous, and you poke your nose before washing your hands, the dangerous substance you had been handling could stick to your nostril and thus breathed in. This then goes straight to the lungs and possibly to the brain too, thus with serious consequences.

The best to do is to use napkin papers or handkerchiefs, and avoid using the already contaminated ones, because they may be worse than poking.

BLOWING YOUR NOSE

When you blow your nose, it is advisable that you use either napkin papers or an handkerchief, because after blowing, there is always a process of cleaning up. In this process of cleaning up, if you happen to use a contaminated napkin paper or an handkerchief, you may end up infecting yourself and thus create more problems for yourself. Literally, you could put germs into your nostrils by using dirty napkin paper or an handkerchief, and the germs or the virus may travel straight into your brain, throat, or even your eyes and cause you major problems.

HAVING SHOWER OR TAKING BATH

REGULARLY

Our bodies always require great attention. We need to care for our bodies on a daily basis. If we neglect to take care of our bodies, they may decay just like any vehicle that is not taken care of, may quickly fall apart.

If we do not wash our bodies on regular basis, they may stink. And this is a total embarrassment to us. This may lead us even to be ostracized by other people. Not that they hate us but simply because of the smell we may be wearing.

In that regard and also to avoid being ostracized by other people, we need to take shower or bath on a regular basis.

Sometimes, if we do not wash our bodies on regular basis, we may develop some diseases, such as scabies, etc.

Washing our bodies is not only for hygiene but it also serves the purpose of therapy or massage. It rejuvenates you, especially hot water when you are just from bed. It gives you new life. Hot water helps in blood circulation and also changing our moods.

Water therapy is very important to our bodies, especially after a day of hard work. It also vanishes the stress you might have had from work or as a result of wrongful association that normally causes us stress.

THE EYES

The eyes are the light to our bodies. They are the natural cameras GOD created in our bodies. They show us what are good and what are bad, what are dangerous and what are not. Besides, they show us the dangers that are ahead of us. Without our eyes, we are under constant darkness.

The eyes also bring you entertainments and therefore make you happy. They help in your education. They help in facilitating the impartation of knowledge. The eyes also protect us from dangerous things, for example, without the eyes, we may fall into deep pits while walking, or step on a dangerous snake etc.

Being one of the most important parts of our bodies, we should always protect them that they may also protect us. There are many ways we could take care of our eyes. These are some of them:

a. Do not rub your eyes

b. Wear protective glasses when doing dangerous job.

a. DO NOT RUB YOUR EYES

Do not rub your eyes because you might rub them with contaminated hands. If you rub your eyes with the hands that were contaminated with dangerous substance, you might become blind instantly. And if you happen to rub your eyes with the hands that are contaminated with germs, you will infect yourself with those germs. You may also cause yourself, sever pains, if you rub your eyes with the hands that were contaminated with hot pepper. The list goes on and on.

b. WEAR PROTECTIVE GLASSES WHEN DOING DANGEROUS JOB

If you doing dangerous job such as welding, working with dangerous chemicals, etc. , you should wear protective glasses in order to avoid becoming blind. If you do not, you are sure to become blind.

THE SOLUTIONS

The solution is never rub your eyes, wash them instead.

And whenever you are going to do dangerous jobs, do not forget to wear your protective glasses.

If you have any eye problem, do not waste time, see the doctor immediately. Any delay to see a doctor, means the situation will worsen, and a simple problem will become more complicated.

CHAPER 2 - WHAT YOU EAT

Have you ever heard the saying, 'We eat to live '? Yeah it is true, we eat to live. Without

food, we can die. Food makes us well and also makes us look good. However, what we eat

may also kill us.

The types of food we eat may determine our health, longevity or premature death.   Of the

types of for we eat, there are those that give us good health and energy, while others that

may totally destroy our health and remove every particle of energy we may have.

Having said all these, we therefore have to be extremely careful of the types of food we eat, if

at all, we want good health and longevity, and also to avoid premature death.

GREASY FOOD

Greasy foods are those foods that are prepared with a lot of cooking oil or fats and other ingredients that make them become greasy. These are considered to be very dangerous foods. They cause obesity. They may also cause high cholesterols to build up in the blood vessels. With the built up of high cholesterols in the blood vessels, they will narrow up and thus restrict the normal blood flow and cause heart attack.

Therefore, if we desire good health, longevity and to avoid premature death, then we should avoid such foods or eat less of them.

FOODS THAT ARE CONTAMINATED

Foods that are contaminated are even more dangerous than greasy foods. Whereas greasy foods may take time to kill you, contaminated foods may kill you instantly. If they do not kill you instantly, they may cause a prolonged health problems, thus making your life, hell on earth. Poor health can prove to be worse than death because your health remains in a daily constant fight for survival, whereas death would do it all at once.

FOODS WITH MORE CHOLESTEROLS

CHAPER 2 - WHAT YOU EAT

Have you ever heard the saying, 'We eat to live'? Yeah it is true, we eat to live. Without food, we can die. Food makes us well and also makes us look good. However, what we eat may also kill us.

The types of food we eat may determine our health, longevity or premature death. Of the types of for we eat, there are those that give us good health and energy, while others that may totally destroy our health and remove every particle of energy we may have.

Having said all these, we therefore have to be extremely careful of the types of food we eat, if at all, we want good health and longevity, and also to avoid premature death.

GREASY FOOD

Greasy foods are those foods that are prepared with a lot of cooking oil or fats and other ingredients that make them become greasy. These are considered to be very dangerous foods. They cause obesity. They may also cause high cholesterols to build up in the blood vessels. With the built up of high cholesterols in the blood vessels, they will narrow up and thus restrict the normal blood flow and cause heart attack.

Therefore, if we desire good health, longevity and to avoid premature death, then we should avoid such foods or eat less of them.

FOODS THAT ARE CONTAMINATED

Foods that are contaminated are even more dangerous than greasy foods. Whereas greasy foods may take time to kill you, contaminated foods may kill you instantly. If they do not kill you instantly, they may cause a prolonged health problems, thus making your life, hell on earth. Poor health can prove to be worse than death because your health remains in a daily constant fight for survival, whereas death would do it all at once.

FOODS WITH MORE CHOLESTEROLS

Foods that have more cholesterols are normally; the pork, the eggs and mayonnaise, etc. Constant steady consumption of these kinds of foods will build in your blood vessels high cholesterols.

Anyway before I go any further, let me remind you that there are two types of cholesterols, the good cholesterols and the bad cholesterols. The good cholesterols are known to be good for our bodies, whereas bad cholesterols are bad for our bodies.

The built up of these bad cholesterols in our bodies that we get from these kinds of foods, will surely cause the narrowing of the blood vessels and possibly heart attacks, just as we saw earlier.

This being the case, and if you like these kinds of foods, eat them in moderation. I eat all these but eat them in moderation. They are very tempting and tasty. And it is their tastes that really lure us to eat them more. Something nice always tend to have firm grip on us, however, if we do not like the pains that might follow or heart attacks, then we should stand our grounds, and say, enough is enough, I am not going to become the victim of your tastes.

FAST FOODS

Fast foods though very tasty, are also classified in the group of foods that cause obesity. Obesity is known to cause serious health problems, from built up cholesterols to less activity of the body. These foods are really not that very bad if only you can eat them in moderation. Realistically, too much of anything even the very best ones, can turn out to be bad and even dangerous. I like the fast food but I know when to say, enough.

And if we go by the now prevailing situation of, this is not good for you, that is not good for you, etc., realistically, then we will have nothing to eat but to starve. I think, moderation of everything is the answer.

PROTECTIVE FOODS

When we talk about protection, everyone seems to want protection. Protection from enemies, protection from accidents, protection from diseases, and the list goes on and on almost endlessly.

And when we talk about protective foods, we are talking about foods that protect us from diseases and other affiliated things.

Protective foods are normally, the fruits and the likes, such as apples, pineapples, oranges, lemons, bananas, vegetables of all kinds, etc.

These foods protect you from diseases and so on. They make your immune system strong to resist any attack from diseases. And these are the foods that will always give you good health and possibly also lead you to longevity.

For the purpose of good health, it is recommended that you eat a given proposed quantity on a daily basis. I know that some of them tend to be very expensive, however, it is not the rule of thumb that you must eat all of them. You may therefore decide to eat one particular type that you like and can easily afford, it really does not matter. All you need is protection and good health. For, where there is health, there is future.

FOOD PREPARATION

Food preparation is as vital as eating the right foods. Eating the right foods leads to good health, equally, eating well and hygienically prepared foods is a prelude to good health also.

However, if you eat good foods but poorly and in hygienically prepared, your quest for good health remains a vanity. A poorly and in hygienically prepared food is not only a symbol of sickness but is as well a symbol of death. Continue to eat such foods and poor health and grave are not far away from you. As the saying goes, ' Prevention is better than cure', so wisely avoid such kinds of foods and such kind of places that prepare such kinds of foods that may send you to the hospitals and may even open the door of the grave for you while you are not yet ready to go there. Be wise, you know the good and the bad, your two eyes are there to help tell you. Do not kill yourself while you still want to live.

AVOID TOO MUCH SMOKY COOKING

Too much smoky cooking is very dangerous to your health. Because the smoke which is normally greasy because of the oil or fats, if inhaled for long time for an extended period, will enter the pores of your lungs and block them, thus cause difficulty in breathing.

Prolonged inhalation of greasy smoke may in long run cause other serious health problems. It may also lead to death because of the blockage. Besides, smoky cooking may seriously affect your kidneys. And if you develop kidney problem, you know that your life may no longer be normal. And a serious kidney problem may require a kidney transplant or else, you may die.

Taking into consideration, the serious problems the smoky cooking may cause, it therefore remains advisable that we should avoid such type of cooking if we want good health and longevity. Alternatively, you should cover the pot to stop smoke from coming out. You should also stay far away from where that kind of cooking is taking place.

CHAPTER 3- WHAT YOU DRINK

What you drink is equally as important as what you eat. It can improve or deteriorate your health. It could also send you early to your grave.

WATER

Water is very essential to our lives. It helps us in washing our bodies, washing our clothes, utensils, preparation of food, drinks, etc. All these are well known to all of us.

Water helps us greatly to keep us healthy. Our bodies require water in order to function normally. We need certain specified amount of water in our bodies for the body to stay healthy. Lack of water in our bodies would cause us dehydration.

Water to our bodies is like gasoline to the vehicles. As the vehicles cannot run without gasoline, so are also our bodies that cannot function normally without water intake.

Besides making the bodies function normally, the intake of water also helps to remove bad odour from within our inner parts. Have you not noticed that after abstaining from water intake, our mouths smell, and this smell comes right from the stomach. Our stomachs can be like a sewage with horrible smell without the water intake.

We also use water for therapy to rejuvenate our bodies. The list of water functions to our bodies is almost endless. Many of these are well known to us.

SOFT DRINKS

Soft drinks are good in taste and sometimes quenching, but may also cause us some serious health problems especially if we do not drink them in moderation.

Too much of soft drinks may cause us to become obsessed. And obesity can lead to other serious health problems, such as diabetics, heart problems.

Constant intake of soft drinks, especially pop drinks, may cause us to have very high level of gas in our stomachs. And very high level of gas in our bodies would cause uneasiness in the bodies. If you have high level of gas in your stomach, you could experience painful attacks running from your stomach to your chest.

Soft drinks can also cause tremendous problems to people with diabetics.

And to avoid all these problems, you should drink soft drinks in moderation, and the diabetics should totally abstain from soft drinks in order to have healthy life.

FRESH JUICE DRINKS

Fresh juice drinks from fruits like oranges, pineapples, apples, etc. are very good for your body. They provide you with protection just like the protection you get from eating the fruits themselves. However, those manufactured with high level of sugar may also be serious problems to people with diabetics. And if you have diabetics, you should be keen to read the labels on the containers and thus avoid buying those manufactured with sugar or high level of sugar. You should buy only those manufactured without sugar.

Water helps us greatly to keep us healthy. Our bodies require water in order to function normally. We need certain specified amount of water in our bodies for the body to stay healthy. Lack of water in our bodies would cause us dehydration.

Water to our bodies is like gasoline to the vehicles. As the vehicles cannot run without gasoline, so are also our bodies that cannot function normally without water intake.

Besides making the bodies function normally, the intake of water also helps to remove bad odour from within our inner parts. Have you not noticed that after abstaining from water intake, our mouths smell, and this smell comes right from the stomach. Our stomachs can be like a sewage with horrible smell without the water intake.

We also use water for therapy to rejuvenate our bodies. The list of water functions to our bodies is almost endless. Many of these are well known to us.

SOFT DRINKS

Soft drinks are good in taste and sometimes quenching, but may also cause us some serious health problems especially if we do not drink them in moderation.

Too much of soft drinks may cause us to become obsessed. And obesity can lead to other serious health problems, such as diabetics, heart problems.

Constant intake of soft drinks, especially pop drinks, may cause us to have very high level of gas in our stomachs. And very high level of gas in our bodies would cause uneasiness in the bodies. If you have high level of gas in your stomach, you could experience painful attacks running from your stomach to your chest.

Soft drinks can also cause tremendous problems to people with diabetics.

And to avoid all these problems, you should drink soft drinks in moderation, and the diabetics should totally abstain from soft drinks in order to have healthy life.

FRESH JUICE DRINKS

Fresh juice drinks from fruits like oranges, pineapples, apples, etc. are very good for your body. They provide you with protection just like the protection you get from eating the fruits themselves. However, those manufactured with high level of sugar may also be serious problems to people with diabetics. And if you have diabetics, you should be keen to read the labels on the containers and thus avoid buying those manufactured with sugar or high level of sugar. You should buy only those manufactured without sugar.

CHAPER 4- THOUGHTS

Thinking is totally unavoidable as long as we live. It is something that GOD ALMIGHTY has

planted in us. We can classify thoughts in two main categories, namely; negative or bad

thoughts and positive or good thoughts. All these have effects on us.

NEGATIVE/BAD THOUGHTS

Negative or bad thoughts can have serious effects on our bodies. They can affect negatively,

the functions of our bodies. And continuous negative thoughts may cause us to become sick.

Even a mere few minutes of serious negative thoughts may cause us, among others, sever headache. Negative thoughts may also affect our appetite.

HOW TO STOP NEGATIVE THOUGHTS

Is it easy to abruptly stop negative thoughts? Yes, it is possible to shut up negative thoughts, but you must program your body to do that. One of the ways, is to switch your thoughts suddenly to something positive or you like. The other way is by repeatedly listening to the music you like. Yet still, you could turn to watching an interesting movie that will fully occupy you up. Other ways would be, starting a conversation with a friend on the same topic or even different topic. Jogging and good environment/scenery is another trick to get rid of negative thoughts. Visualizing something with possible terrible consequences of the negative thoughts may also help you to stop that negative thought. Visualize the heart problem you may have, visualize the paralysis of your body that may come about because of this negative thought. Visualize the helplessness that you will be in should you become chronically ill because of this negative thought.

And once your brain comes to grip with all these visualizations, it will cut in and shut off the negative thoughts, and immediately.

POSITIVE THOUGHTS

Positive thoughts are good for our bodies. They make us feel good about ourselves and also boost up our self- esteems. Besides, they can bring progress in our lives. Yet still, they help in keeping our health in good shape because we are happy and the body is at peace.

Positive thoughts may also wet up our appetite. And when we eat well, that is definitely good for our health.

WORRIES

We can be our worst enemies by indulging ourselves into worries. Worries can seriously deprive you peace of mind. They may also send you to hospitals. Worries can cause us quite a number of problems and will adversely affect our health.

These are some of the problems worrying may cause you:

1. Depression

2. Loss of weight

3. Heart problem

4. Stroke

5. Aggression

6. Suicide

7. Stomach problems, such as constipation, ulcer, etc.

8. Headache

9. Migraine

10. Hypertension, etc.

11. Worrying may also send you prematurely to your grave.

SOLUTIONS

a. Some of the solutions in stopping negative thoughts, also work for `worries.

b. Realize that by worrying, you cannot solve the problem, but will create more problems.

c. Recollect the number of people who you know who by worrying a lot, have caused themselves problems such as heart attacks, depression, stroke, etc.

d. Visualize how you may become a complete vegetable and have to depend on other people as a result of worrying a lot.

e. Also think of the sufferings that you will cause to your family in case you become disabled.

f. Get engaged into doing something that will fully occupy you and leave you no time for worrying.

g. Be in a company of positive and good friends.

h. Seek for professional advice.

i. In case the worrying persists, see the doctor. You never know it could turn out to be a mental problem, because some people worry over nothing.

CHAPTER 5- EXERCISES

Regular exercises will always cause us to be healthy. And lack of exercises may do exactly the opposite. Lack of exercises will cause us to be sick in many ways.

Some of the problems lack of exercises may bring on us are:

1. **OBESITY**

   Because of lack of exercises, we may become obsessed. And we have already looked at the problems that obesity may cause us.

2. **HEART PROBLEMS**

By being totally idle without doing exercises, and accompanied by obesity, we may also develop heart problems.

3. HIGH BLOOD PRESSURE

If your body is not exercised regularly, you may also end up developing high blood pressure. And you know what problems come with this. We already looked at some of these problems.

4. DIABETICS

Because of lack of exercises and the weight you have gained, you may end up with diabetics. And diabetics is a complete nuisance that will turn your life around. It will also deprive you a lot of things, such as not eating sweet things, it may also affect your sexual functions, etc.

5. LAZINESS

As you idle yourself, you may become very fat and this may lead you to become very lazy. And laziness can also generate a lot of other problems, such as poverty, sickness, etc.

6. JOGGING

You can remain fit when you decide to jog at least few hours every week. This will make your body function normally and you also remain healthy.

7. WALKING

Walking is also another form of exercise. By taking a walk everyday or few days a week, you are giving your body the exercise it needs.

8. SWIMMING

Swimming is yet another form of exercise that makes your body healthy. It also makes you to become mentally alert.

9. CYCLING

When you cycle, you are doing a tremendous exercise, especially when you peddle uphill or put your gear to high one. Cycling will keep you fit.

10. **DANCING**

Dancing too is a form of exercise. And the good thing with dancing is that you enjoy it. That therefore means you are shooting two birds with one stone. One is the enjoyment derivation and the other, is the exercise itself.

11. **THE GYM**

The gym will give you all forms of exercises. As you go from one form of exercise to another, your body will immensely benefit and also remain fit.

WHAT EXERCISES CAN DO TO YOUR BODY

There are a lot of good things, exercises can give your body. Some of these are:

1. Exercise can fight the disease in your body.

2. Exercise will fight obesity.

3. Exercise will make you mentally alert.

4. Exercise will boost up your immune system.

5. Exercise can make you have the shape of body you want.

6. Exercise can make your skin smooth, shinny and healthy.

7. Exercise can boost up your sexual functions and desires.

8. Exercise can cause normal blood circulation in your body.

9. Exercise will strengthen your bones.

10. Exercise will boost up your appetite.

11. Exercise will extend your lifespan, in other words gives you longevity.

CHAPTER 6- YOUR FAMILY, RELATIVES AND OTHER PEOPLE

It is definitely a blessing to have a family and relatives. They are there to help in many ways. In things that you are totally unable to handle and solve, they are there to give you a helping hand. And they care more than anybody else because you are a part of them.

It is their joy when you are okay. They also know well enough that in case of problems, your help may also be there for them. It is scratch my back and I will scratch yours situation. And this the normal norm in any family that functions normally.

However, there are families that unnecessarily normally tear themselves apart. They never co-operate with one another. And they look at the fall of a family member as a joy and a success for them. Such families are full of jealousy and hatred. They never want anyone else in the family to succeed.

This is totally an absurd situation and near to nothing else, but a curse. Can such a situation be changed? Of course yes, for there is no problem without a solution. The change can start with you and spread over to every member of the family. You need to turn your back to hatred and jealousy. You also need to start to sincerely forgive any member of the family that has done you wrong intentionally and unintentionally. Know that you are knitted together by GOD for a purpose, and it is not an accident. Besides, you need to practise kindness and to be happy at the success of any family member.

Build a paradise in your home, for it is the only place that should give you joy, peace and protections from the world's beatings. Be the first to change your family and have a healthy living that comes out of happiness.

PROBLEMS THAT CAN ARISE IN NON-CO-OPERATING FAMILIES

If a family has deliberately refused to be a family, there could arise a lot of problems. And these are some of the problems that may arise:

a. There can always be the quarrels in the family.

b. There could also be fights in the family.

c. There could also arise injuries to family members as results of the fights.

d. As quarrels and fights go on unabated, there could also arise arrests and imprisonments.

e. There will never be any progress in that family.

f. There will be under development and deteriorating situations in the family.

g. There may also arise manipulations of the family by the outsiders because the happen to know everything about the family.

h. Continuous misunderstandings may cause some family members to become sick.

i. And continuous fights unfortunately, one day lead to the death of a family member.

j. A bad family member may also one day betray the family and thus lead to the demise of that family.

k. Consistent quarrels, fights and misunderstandings may lead to total destruction of that family, in the form of separation, divorce, etc.

l. This kind of awkward lifestyle, will always deprive you happiness, good health and totally deny you longevity. In other words, it may send you early to your grave.

As I said earlier, there is no problem without a solution, and surely, if you are determined to solve the misunderstandings in your family, you definitely can.

The first step is to become another you and begin to radiate changes and understandings in the family. There are several things you could do to arrest a bad situation in your family. And some of these are:

1. Change yourself, become a peacemaker.

2. Learn to forgive even if you are deeply hurt by a family member.

3. Work hard to change any situation that may be causing misunderstanding.

4. Visualize the untold problems that you could cause your family members. If you do not enjoy it, then shut the door to that thing that causes you to hurt others.

5. Realize that you could also become the victim.

6. Feel the pains other family members are going through.

7. Realize that by following the trend of misunderstandings, the family will never progress as it embarks on nothing else but fully occupy with everyday problems solving.

8. Also realize that by continuous having misunderstandings, you are going to cause a death of a family member.

9. Sincerely and openly discuss any problem in the family.

OTHER RELATIVES

Relatives are relatives whether we like or not and we cannot in any way change that. However, there are some relatives who would work for your downfall. And there are others who could turn out to be real thorns in your flesh. While others who are fully obsessed with jealousy and never want you to succeed in life.

WHAT TO DO

If you know that there are relatives who are bad to you, and may cause you problems, cut them off from your life and spare yourself not only a headache but also health problems.

OTHER PEOPLE

Do not allow other people to cause you headaches and problems. Keep the good ones and get rid of the bad ones. If you allow the bad ones to stick to you, they will cause you untold problems and sufferings. Remember, they do not care a bit for your fall is their achievement, your pains their happiness and your sufferings, their celebrations. Keep them away. You can live without them. Have you never lived without them before? Do not be fooled and do not

fool yourself. Get back your peace of mind and be healthy.

CHAPTER 7- DOMESTIC ENVIRONMENT

When we talk of domestic environment, we are virtually talking about things such as

washrooms, or toilet sanitation, kitchen sanitation, the human interactions environments.

At this particular moment, I will dwell on sanitation as human environment will be dealt with

later on.

Some of these have already partially been dealt with. Let us therefore now look at such things

as kitchen sanitation and washroom sanitation. These are actually the most important places

in a house. Poor upkeep of these two places in any house denotes possible serious problems.

Let us start with the kitchen.

KITCHEN SANITATION AND POSSIBLE PROBLEMS

Kitchen sanitation is possibly the most important when it comes to hygiene. Why is it so important? Because what you eat is prepared there.

When a kitchen is kept clean is a prelude to good health. Because the food that is prepared there is not possibly contaminated, and therefore provides healthy eating. Whereas if a kitchen is not kept clean it may cause us some serious health problems later on.

Firstly, because it is not looked after well and is dirty, may end up attracting flies that may bring germs to the food that is already prepared, or to the foodstuffs that are yet to be prepared. Knowing what the flies are, they may not only bring the germs but also some other contaminants.

The dirty kitchen may also breed cockroaches. And cockroaches are another form of nuisance and germs and disease transmitters. They run around and land and feed on anything including the food that you may eat. Inevitably, this becomes the source of sickness and disease contraction.

Yet, there may be other forms of contamination due the dirt that clings around the kitchen. Dirty kitchen may also attract mice into the house and particularly the kitchen. They are attracted by the staunch of food that we leave around uncovered. And mice can bring us a lot of health problems including rabies.

To avoid all these problems, we should always keep our kitchens clean. And we should not let the food that we do not need hang around exposed. We should wrap them up. And if we are using the bins, we should make sure that we empty them frequently. If we are not yet ready to empty them, then we should cover them up.

Besides, we should clean the kitchen after every cooking and wash all the utensils and the cutleries immediately after we have finished eating. Leaving utensils, plates and the cutleries that we have used, unwashed will attract these unwanted intruders.

WASHROOMS

Washrooms are another important places in a house. It is in the washrooms that the germs normally breed and thus spread to the whole house. This may cause us to become sick and also attract the disease that may cause us serious health problems and make us miserable for the rest of our lives.

BEDROOMS

It is also important that we keep our bedrooms tidy all the time. We should regularly wash our bedsheets, blankets and pajamas to avoid breeding lice and bedbugs which are a complete nuisance and an embarrassment.

AIR FRESHENERS

Air fresheners are very good for fighting the odour that makes the place to stink and also makes our lives miserable. However, too much of air freshener could also turn out to be a health hazard.

And if you decide to use air freshener, use it in moderation in order not to affect your health.

INSECTICIDE

Insecticides are poison. They may not only kill the insects and the bugs, but may also kill you especially if you inhale it for a long time.

When you decide to spray your home with an insecticide, make sure that you wear a mask to protect you from inhaling it. And after spraying, leave the house immediately for at least some hours. Come back in the house when you know that everything has settled down.

And when you come back after hours of staying away from your house, open all the windows for the smell to go out. Clean thoroughly all the places in the house to get rid of the settled insecticide.

Remember, long breading of insecticide will affect your lungs and may cause breathing difficulty. It may also cause immediate headache and throat problems. Besides, it may also affect your kidneys.

PRIOR TO SPRAYING

Before spraying the house, you must make sure that you store away in a safe place, the food, foodstuffs, the utensils, plates, cutleries, etc. to avoid them being contaminated.

DETERGENTS

Dish washing liquid is good for cleaning our utensils, plates, etc. but it could also turn out to be a mild poison that may kill us later on, especially after a prolonged use. And moreover, washing of utensils, cutleries, etc. may not be only once in a day. It could be numerous times in a day. And this is a real threat to our health. It becomes even more dangerous when we use hot water. With hot water, the steam that comes out and we inhale, is fully saturated with this mild and slow killing poison.

AVOIDANCE

The way to avoid poisoning ourselves with this mild poison, is to use dishwashing machines if we can afford. However, not everyone can afford dishwashers.

The affordable and effective way is to use cold water. With cold water, there is no steam, there is only the smell and therefore we are free from inhaling this toxin.

PERFUMES

Some perfumes give really good smell but there are others with very horrible smell.

Regardless of the smell, perfumes are also a kind of poison. You could call them mild poison.

Prolonged use of perfumes may in the long run cause serious health problems. Therefore, use them in moderation to avoid suffering later on.

GENERAL CLEANING

Hygienically it is important that we should clean our houses everyday in order to get rid of the germs and bacteria. If we do not clean our houses often, they become dirty, and dust also quickly settles on almost everything in the house. In the dust, there could be bacteria and germs. And when we inhale this contaminated dust, we fall sick. And often sickness is almost a roadblock to longevity.

THE SHOES

The shoes are literally meant to protect our feet from things that may hurt them. They are also meant to protect our feet from germs and other related things.

Shoes though are mean to protect us from various things, might also turn out to be the real source of critical health problems. Shoes step on many undesirable things as we walk. Just to name a few, the step on dog poops, spits, cough spits, etc. and if we just walk into our houses, right into the kitchen, living room, bedrooms, etc. without removing them, we may carry quite dangerous things to those places. And these dangerous things will later on turn to be our nightmares.

SOLUTIONS

1. Make sure to remove your shoes just at the door when you come from outside.

2. Regularly clean and disinfect the place that you use for storing your shoes.

3. Occasionally, wash and disinfect your shoes, those that are not leather. The leather ones you could merely disinfect.

CHAPTER 8- EXTERNAL

ENVIRONMENTS

Outside environment is normally polluted with different kinds of pollutions, ranging from cigarette smoke to vehicle smoke. All these are a disaster to our health.

CIGARETTE SMOKE

Cigarette smoke is by far the most dangerous and a quiet killer. Cigarette smoke is also by far has killed more people than the atomic bombs have done. It kills without discrimination, both the smokers and non-smokers.

Smoke from cigarettes are known to cause a lot of health problems, such as heart disease, cancer, stroke, etc. Definitely, there could be many more problems cigarette smoke can cause. The sad part of it is that it affects even those that hate smoking. It is totally unfair, it is like you are being poisoned. Second hand smoke is known to be even worse. Are there ways one could avoid this? Yes, there are of course some ways. A few are appended below.

HOW TO STAY AWAY FROM THIS DEADLY SMOKE

1. Avoid a place where people are smoking.

2. Do not associate with those who smoke since they appear to have no control over their bad habit and smoke anywhere, regardless.

3. Where smoking is taking place, be it on the street or anywhere else, avoid the direction of the wind.

These are the few things you could do to avoid be killed by this unwanted smoke. And there is no reason why people should smoke, when repeatedly, they are warned of the dangers of dying from this killer smoke.

VEHICLE SMOKE

Vehicle smoke can prove to be very fatal if inhaled for a long time. It contains carbon dioxide. And carbon dioxide is toxic. If you happen to inhale it for a long time, you can collapse, have immediate headache, chest pains, etc.

As a prevention measure, always avoid the direction of the wind. This will stop you from inhaling this toxic and dangerous smoke.

If you are jogging or walking, always be on the opposite side of the wind direction. Alternatively, choose to jog or walk on the road that has no or less traffic.

DRUG SMOKE

The smoke of any drug that you may accidentally inhale puts you at risk equally with the one who is smoking it. And continuous inhalation of this smoke may seriously cause you serious health problems. Though innocent, you may eventually become mad like the drug users themselves. You may in the long run become a vegetable, at worst, you may also become violent and ready to commit crimes.

AVOIDANCE

1. At all costs, stay away from drug users in order to save your health and life.
2. Avoid places that are infested by the drug users.
3. If you notice or feel the smell of any drug, avoid the direction of the wind.
4. On public transport, if you feel anybody with drug smell, move away, because that smell alone will seriously affect you after breathing it for long.
5. If you are renting in a place that has drug users, quickly relocate before it is too late.

And lastly, do not smoke or use drugs of any kind, they will merely destroy you and slowly kill you.

FACTORY SMOKE

If you live near a factory or factories, consider relocation. If you take it easy and do not work out an appropriate and a preventive solution, you may in the long run develop some health issues, such as cancer, heart problem, kidney problems, etc. because of the continuous inhalation of the toxic chemicals.

And if you happen to work in any one of them, always remember to wear a mask.

WHISTLING IN A DIRTY PLACE WHILE DOING A DIRTY JOB

To whistle in a dirty place where you are doing a dirty job and where dangerous chemicals are kept, or in a factory where the spills of toxic chemicals may contaminate the air, means an invitation to serious health problems.

Because by whistling in such places, you are actually sucking the chemicals or the poison, etc. right into your lungs. And the flow of these chemicals or the poison into your lungs are very forceful and rapid because of the power of the whistle. Within a short time it might overcome you and if not rushed to the hospital immediately, you might even die.

So the advice is, avoid at all costs, whistling in dirty places or when you are doing a dirty job in order to avoid health problems or even shortening your life.

CHAPTER 9- SEX

Sex as we all know it is good to everyone. Apart from the purpose of multiplication, sex also gives us pleasure. However, we have to be extremely careful with whom we are going to have sex. In most religions, one is not supposed to have sex before marriage. And sex outside marriage is totally forbidden by GOD ALMIGHTY. To do so is to sin. This is one of The Ten Commandments of GOD, thou shall not commit adultery.

CARELESS SEX

To have sex with anybody is not only degrading but is also a source of disease contraction. If you are involved in careless sex, you should know that you are prone to many diseases such as gonorrhea, syphilis, aids, etc.

Any of these diseases that you may contract may ruin your health, sometimes, may lead even to death. Aids in particular is a very deadly disease that can kill you. At this moment of time, aids has no cure but can merely be controlled to a certain extent.

WICKED SPOUSE

A wicked spouse is a very dangerous partner who may cause you untold sufferings. He or she may not only make you hurt by other people but may also infect you with one of those deadly sexual diseases. Besides, he or she may make you hurt other people, if they do not hurt you. You may also go to prison because of a wicked spouse.

In addition to the above, a wicked spouse remains also a danger to your children. Your children may be born with one of those diseases. And this may ruin their entire lives.

PROTECTED SEX

These days the use of condoms have become the order of the day. Yes, condoms may protect but you never know when they may rapture. And in the case of rapture, you may automatically be exposed to any of these dangers. The diseases that you were trying to protect yourself from, immediate become in full control.

Not only the rapture can occur but sometimes, the condom may just slip off because it was not fitted well due to the size. If this occurs, you are not only exposed to the diseases but the condom may also remain deep inside your partner and that may require the help of a medical doctor to take it out, or else it may later on cause a major health problem to one in whom it has remained.

Although people have resorted to use condoms as the means of protection from these sexual diseases, yet they may not give us a complete protection that we want, because of the following reasons:

1. The condom may rapture during the course of intercourse.
2. The condom may slip into the vagina and thus leaving you totally exposed to any of these diseases.
3. The remains of the semen in the body may become a cause of concern.

THE BEST CONTROL

The best way to avoid all these sexual problems, is to abstain from sex if possible. Secondly, avoid being like an animal whereby you become a prey to everyone. Yet still, have sex only with your partner.

Unfortunately, in the case of a partner, you cannot even be sure that you are safe especially when you have a bad partner and an animal like. And if you happen to know that your partner is a free for all partner, the best solution in this case is to get rid of her or him to be on the safe side. Otherwise, you are fully exposed to all kinds of dangers and you do not know when they may strike.

TREATMENT

If you happen to acquire any of these diseases, seek treatment immediately. In your course of treatment, do not hide anything like some other people may do, be frank to the doctor and tell him or her the exact problem that you may get the right treatment. If you do not reveal your exact problem, then you may decay. If you have gonorrhea, do not tell a doctor that you have a severe headache, just because you are ashamed to reveal the truth. And if you do, you will be given the medication for headache instead for gonorrhea. This is not only stupid but is more so a serious danger to your life.

While undergoing treatment, do not sex with other people because you may spread the disease. Temporarily, abstain yourself from sex.

CHAPTER 10- AVOID STRESSFUL LIFE

Stress is not only dangerous but is also a killer. If you allow stress to take over your life, then happiness will totally depart from you and unhappiness will set in, thus upsetting your life altogether and make you to live a complete life of misery and torture.

Remember, stress has mercy for anyone. It attacks anybody anytime and anywhere without prior warning. It will come with numerous problems to decay and totally destroy your body. The accompaniments could range from:

a. Depression

b. Chest pains

c. Hypertension

d. Stomach upset and pains

e. Loss of appetite

f. Heart attack

g. Stroke

h. Craziness

i. Isolation, to much more serious problems.

DEPRESSION

As a result of stress, if you acquire depression, your life will become a torture. You will not be happy in life. Your mind will wonder from one problem to another, including things that merely imaginary. You may also develop the spirit of fear.

Depression is a very disturbing and a wild disease that is very difficult to get rid of once contracted. The only best medicine for it, is never to contract it in the first place. And not to contract it, is to stay away from stressful life.

CHEST PAINS

Chest pains is not only a nuisance but it is so cruel that can make your life totally miserable. When you have the chest pains, you can at times become unable to do anything. The pain can be really bad and may take a while before getting better. The sad part is that, a continuous chest pains may eventually lead to heart problems.

HYPERTENSION

Hypertension is yet another child of the stress. It is another complicated health problem that require constant taking of medication to control it.

The best solution is not to acquire it. That means staying away from stressful life and other things that cause it.

STOMACH UPSET AND PAINS

Because of stress, you may have occasional stomach upsets and pains. These can make your life very miserable and occasionally, you may need medication to control it.

LOSS OF APPETITE

Stressful life may also cause you loss of appetite. You may not even be able to enjoy the food that you like.

HEART ATTACK

Because of constant pressure on the heart, you may end up having heart attack. And heart attack may instantly end up your life when you are not yet ready to go. And if you happen to survive it, you may become a vegetable with inability to do anything in your life. You will become a total dependant on other people.

This being the case so hard to swallow, you should therefore avoid stressful life all together. If you begin to feel that stress is invading your life, immediately remind yourself of the possible consequences and the aftermaths. With this step you have taken, also immediately curtail any invading negative thoughts.

STROKE

When you have a stroke as a result of stress, you may become temporarily or permanently paralyzed. And this will have serious consequences in your life as you become unable to do anything in your life. You will need people to depend on as you may not be able to move or even lift your hands. Your brain and your speech may also become seriously affected. You want be able to think logically and your memories may become completely impaired. This becomes not just a mere torture, but it is also a near death type of life as you struggle to live.

CRAZINESS

Stress may also cause you to become literally crazy. And if you develop a serious mental problem, then you are finished unless GOD helps you. If by the grace of GOD you recover, then that is your luck and miracle. If you bank your hope in Mental Hospital, that is a total vanity as many of the patients from there end up worse than they went in. Besides, there are so many issues with Mental Hospitals.

ISOLATION

Because stress, you might consciously or unconsciously decide to isolate yourself from other people as you become dreadful of everything and every environment. While it may protect you from bad people and bad things, it is also a serious problem of its own.

SOLUTIONS

Since this is by far a dangerous monster, you therefore need to run away from it as fast as possible. And as there are virtually solutions to all problems, stress is not an exception. Stress like any other problems, has solutions. And below are some of the solutions that may fight stress. These are:

1. BE HAPPY

By being happy, you are bombarding the stress with your deadly weapon and keeping it away from you. And when you are happy, your body functions normally. By the body normal function, diseases and sickness are also kept away. This also enables the body to increase the immune system that may fight any invading force.

2. LISTEN TO THE MUSIC THAT MAKES YOU HAPPY

Whenever the stress is preparing to invade you, turn on the music that you like and make you happy. Listen to it repeatedly until you have regained your normal mind. This way, you are actually removing your mind away from what is stressing you up. And by concentrating into your music, you derive happiness and forget whatever was stressing you out.

WATCH THE MOVIE YOU LIKE

Watching the movie that you like has the same tricks like listening to the music you like. When you give no time to stress to bother you by watching the movie you like, you are not only giving it a warning but killing it. And as you concentrate into watching and with some parts of the movie that bring you laughter, the stress begins to retreat and eventually disappear into the blues.

LAUGHTER

Laughter brightens not only your face but also your heart and eliminates so many bad things from your body. This must not be cosmetic but real laughter from things that are funny or make you happy and laugh.

DO THE JOB YOU ENJOY TO DO

Some jobs can be very stressful, especially those you do not like but simply do it in order to make money. These kinds of jobs will eventually cause you, health problems in long run.

Also a bad boss may cause you serious stress and ruin your health.

Health is very important to everyone. We are able to generate money when we are healthy, and if we are unhealthy, we become unable to work and the follow of money may cease too. This may also means a lot of more other problems.

In that regard, if your work stresses you out, quit it and look for another one. Equally, if you have a boss who is always on your neck, say bye to him, it is better to be healthy than cling on to that money source that tears you apart everyday. However, if you insist and continue, it is not only your health that is endangered but your life-span is also being shortened.

LET NOTHING BOTHER YOU

We are our own enemies in many ways. We ignorantly allow bad thoughts to infiltrate our minds and cause us stress and consequently cause also poor health. As if the problems we might be having are not enough, we further go on to worry over things that may not even happen. We also allow other people to invade our minds and cause us serious stress. And if there is really a bad situation, take note, even this will pass away as nothing is forever. Be happy. You may say, 'How can I be happy with all these problems that surround me?' I have just told you, even this will pass away for nothing is forever. Had you no problems in the past? And are they still there? Then why worry over something that will eventually go away? Remember, there is none under the sky without problems. Your health is more important than the worries you are carrying.

DON'T LET BAD THINGS CLING INTO YOUR HEAD

The sure way not to get stressed out is not to allow bad thoughts, feelings, etc. cling into your head for an extended period of time. Do you know how the iron becomes bendable? The pressure of constant fire will make this unbendable iron bendable.

And by clinging in your head, the bad feelings, thoughts or bad things that have occurred, you are virtually putting your body under intensive pressure and eventually that body will bend, and you suffer the consequences.

CHAPTER 11- TREATMENTS

We all become sick one time or the other. Different things and environments may send us sick sometimes when we least expect it. However, we must always work hard to recover from whatever sickness. And the sure way to quickly recover, is to immediately seek treatments.

We should not waste time when we become sick, because, time wasted may mean deterioration of our condition. And we do not want that to happen to us because good health is very important. With good health, we are able to accomplish a lot of things, but when we are sick, we become totally unable to accomplish even the least.

TREATMENTS

If you become sick, seek immediate medical attention. In seeking treatments, you should be frank with the doctors, and always call a spade, a spade and never hide your disease because of shame. If you do, you will not get cured because you will be given wrong medication while your body continue to rot. This is more so with sexual diseases. Many people tend to hide them because of shame. One might have contracted syphilis for example, and when with a doctor for the history of the sickness, will say, 'I have a severe headache'. And the doctor will therefore prescribe the medicine for headache, while the guy remains rotting. And when he or she is out of the clinic, will say to himself or herself, 'This doctor is very stupid, I will never come back to this clinic'. The question remains, who is stupid here, the doctor or you?

Be frank, tell the doctor the actual sickness that you may get the right treatment. This is normal, everybody gets sick at one time or the other. Sometimes may be with these shameful diseases. So what? Just do not be ashamed, you never know, may be this doctor also one time had the same problem. It is the question of a partner.

FOLLOWING THE RULES OF MEDICATION

If the doctor prescribes for you some medication, it is extremely essential that you adhere to the rules therein. To get cured, you should always follow the instructions given to you by the doctor. And make sure that you finish the medication even if you happen to get better before the medicine is finished.

In giving you the medication, the doctors know that for the disease to be totally eradicated from your body, the medicine must be completely finished and within the specified time.

Some people when they begin to feel better, abandon taking the medication. And this is totally wrong, because the disease may recur as it was merely drowsy and not yet fully conquered.

While others, instead of finishing the medication within the specified time, will prolong the period, and thus weakens the treatment and reinforces the disease. This too is wrong. If you really want to be cured, finish the medication within the specified period and also stick to the times, you were told to be taking this medication. Do not come up with your own program for you are not a doctor, and if you were, then there would have been no need for you to go to that doctor. Do not fool yourself if you want to get better.

And if a doctor tells you not to do certain things while on medication, follow it for there is a reason behind it.

OVERDOSE

Worst still, there some people when a doctor recommends to them to take a given quantity per day, they overlook that and want to take more quantity in order to get cured quickly. This is very dangerous. By doing so, you are just going to kill yourself. The doctor knows that too much of that is fatal that is why he or she instructs you to stick to the prescribed quantity.

TRANSFERRING THE MEDICATION

Yet still, there are people who when they are given the medication, they then immediately also become the doctors without training, to another who may be sick. They will give the medication that they were given to another person, to treat him or her, and not knowing that the medication was given to particularly treat the disease he or she has.

This is a huge problem. The transfer of such medication may cause enormous problems to the recipient. You may also end up killing that person. And if should this happen, you can be charged with manslaughter.

SAFE KEEPING OF MEDICATION

Safe keeping of medication, means complete protection. As important as it is, you should always keep your medication in safe places, away from children who may accidentally or inquisitively take them. Also remember to mark medication containers or bottles, so you know which is for which and for who.

Besides, for other medication that you buy over the counter, always remember to take note of the expiration dates, because some medicine may automatically become poisonous after they expire. And some of them may lose their power of cure.

VITAMINS

Vitamin supplements are good for our bodies. They supplement what we may lack from the natural sources. Take them regularly to protect you and to provide you good health. Again, do not overdose yourself. Always go by the instructions on the containers. Play safe and avoid dangers.

AVOID CONTAMINATED MEDICINE

Always avoid the medicine that is contaminated. Let us say if the medicine falls down on the floor while you are taking it, do not swallow that one any more. If you decide to take it, you may infect yourself with some other diseases, and increase more health problems to your body.

Or if you store your medication in a place that can easily contaminate it, if you notice of any contamination, throw that medication away. Do not take it, thinking that it may still work, no, just throw it away. And if you take it, you will simply be poisoning yourself.

CHAPTER 12- DRINK BUT IN

MODERATION

Drinking is not a sin and will never be a sin. GOD ALMIGHTY did not classify the drinking of alcohol as a sin. HE never said, 'Thou shall not drink'.

The reasons why some of the religions do not permit drinking is because, drinking can breed sins in some people when they become drunk. They may commit sins under intoxication. And the commission of the sins may happen unconsciously. So is also the commission of crimes under intoxication, but to purposely drink in order to commit sins or crime is inexcusable. Because this is intended or has what the law call malice aforethought. And with that kind of mind, you are never free of your action.

REACTIONS TO DRINKS

Some people become so happy when they drink, while others become aggressive and even miserable.

You therefore have to find out in which category you fall whenever you drink. Are you happy when you drink, or are you aggressive and depressed whenever you drink?

If the drinks make you happy and eliminate your stress, then go for them, alternatively, if they make you miserable and depressed, then you need to quit before you put yourself into terrible troubles.

PROBLEMS THAT DRINKS CAN CAUSE YOU

Drinks can cause one a number of problems. Some of these are:

a. If drinks make you aggressive, you may fight.

b. If drinks make you aggressive, you may hurt someone.

c. If drinks make you aggressive and miserable and aggressive, you may kill.

d. If drinks make you aggressive and overexcited, you may rape someone.

e. If drinks make you aggressive, you may one day go to jail.

f. If drinks make you aggressive, you may one day be hurt by someone.

g. If drinks make you aggressive, you may one day be killed by someone.

h. If drinks make you sad, you may one day commit suicide.

i. If drinks aggressive, they may one day cause a separation or even a divorce in your family.

j. Drinks may also make you hurt yourself.

k. Overdrinking may kill you.

l. Drinks may cause hangover and severe headache.

GOOD SIDES OF DRINKS

Some drinks are medicinal, they may treat certain ailments in your body. Drinks in most cases temporarily remove stress from our bodies. They also permit rapid normal circulation of blood in our bodies.

Wine in particular is recommended for good health. Again, do not abuse it, but drink in moderation.

CHAPTER 13- DO NOT SMOKE

People who smoke are prone to a lot of health issues. Some of these health issues we have already looked at them. However, to drive the point home, we will look at them again.

The problems that smoking cigarettes may cause you are:

1. LUNG CANCER

    Because of smoking, you may develop lung cancer.

2. THROAT CANCER

    Smoking may also cause you to have throat cancer.

3. **HEART DISEASE**

Your continuous smoking may also bring you heart disease.

4. **CANCER OF THE MOUTH**

You may also end up with cancer of the mouth because of smoking cigarettes.

Yet still, there are so many other problems that smoking can cause you. And some

of these problems are:

a. **LIFE-SPAN**

Smoking can shorten your life-span.

b. **YOUR FAMILY**

Smoking may also cause you your family. If your family members do

not smoke and do not like smoke, your perpetual smoking may

disintegrate the family.

c. **FRIENDS**

Smoking may cause you friends. If your friends do not smoke and hate

smoke, they may decide to quit the friendship for their health.

d. **DEATH**

Your continuous smoking in the house may kill members of your family, or

even yourself. You may also cause the deaths of other people as you continue

to smoke in places, on the streets, etc.

e. **SICKNESS**

By persistently smoking in the house, you may cause your family members to

contract diseases, such as, heart disease, cancer, stroke, etc. You may also

affect other people.

f. LEGAL ISSUES

Smoking may also cause you legal issues.

QUIT SMOKING AND SAVE YOUR LIFE AND THE LIVES OF OTHER PEOPLE

When you finally decide to quit smoking, you are doing yourself and other people, a favour.

Quitting is always not easy, but where there is a will, there is always the possibility. And there are so many means to quit smoking, one of them is Nicorette. Besides Nicorette, there are many others

CHAPTER 14- AVOID DRUGS

Drugs can not only cause you health issues, but they also set you against authorities. Drugs are contrabands, in other words, they are illegal. They can cause you a lot of problems. Some of these problems are:

1. Drug can turn you into a vegetable.

2. Drugs will destroy your brain.

3. Drugs will cause you madness.

4. Drugs will cause you to become aggressive.

5. Drugs can cause you to injure other people.

6. Drugs can cause you to kill other people.

7. Drugs can send you to prison.

8. Drugs can cause you to be killed by other drug users or peddlers.

9. In some other countries, such in many Asian countries, you can be killed by firing squad.

10. Because of drugs, you may also lose your family.

11. Your friends may also desert you.

12. Because of drugs you may become a wanted person by the authorities.

13. Drugs will totally destroy your entire health.

14. Drugs will shorten your life-span and you die a premature death.

SOLUTION

Just stay away from all forms of drugs.

CHAPTER 15- SLEEP

Sleep forms part of our lives. It is very essential for the normal body function. Sleep also recuperates our bodies from the exhaustion of the day's work. It is the body's garage where the body undergoes maintenance on a nightly or daily basis.

SLEEP DEPRIVATION

Sleep deprivation can cause us a lot of problems. If you deprive your body from sleep, you may witness the following:

1. Lack of sleep may cause you dizziness.

2. Lack of sleep may cause weakness in the body.

3. Lack of sleep may cause you an accident when you are driving.

4. Lack of sleep may make you become aggressive.

5. Lack of sleep will deprive you concentration.

6. Lack of sleep will cause a headache.

7. Lack of sleep will interrupt the normal function of the body.

8. If you happen to develop insomnia, you may become stressed out, due to the fact that your mind will wonder from one problem to another. And opening different chapters of your problems as the sleep escapes you. By the time morning turns in, you are already depressed.

9. Lack of sleep may also cause you to have an accident or even be killed when you work in a factory and operate a dangerous machine.

10. Lack of sleep may also strain your eyesight.

11. And lack of sleep may also age you very fast.

These are the few of the many problems lack of sleep can cause one.

HAVING ENOUGH SLEEP

When you have enough sleep, your body is at peace. It makes your body to function normally. Besides, it brings joy in your heart. And when you are asleep that is when the maintenance of your body takes place. This is comparative to the maintenance of the buses that undergo daily maintenance after a day of running around, and are made ready for another day. In the sleep is when recuperation of the body also takes place.

Sleep also fights stress effectively. Because when you are asleep, you stay away from the problems that bother you. Besides, sleep rejuvenates you, and you stay young. It is due to the fact that at that time, your body is totally free from worries and things that bother you as we have just seen.

Another top secret of the sleep, is that it is a rehearsal of what is to come, death. It is GOD's secret reminder to us, that whatever may be, death awaits you. Don't let this bother you though, it is just the secret of GOD ALMIGHTY.

IF YOU HAVE INSOMNIA

When you develop insomnia, and it has become persistent, it is better to see a doctor in order to diagnose the problem and arrive at a solution. And there are certain things in life that might cause us insomnia including the things we drink and eat. Too much coffee taking especially when you are about to go to bed, may cause you lack of sleep. Some people are also affected by tea, tea deprives them of sleep. Another thing is that, they might have too many worries in their chapters, and keep on flipping pages after pages of their problems. Also another thing that may cause us lack of sleep, are the pains we might have. If your body is in serious pain, surely you cannot sleep.

SOLUTIONS

1. Make sure that you see a doctor to treat that insomnia.

2. Reduce your coffee intake especially when going to bed.

3. If you are one of those affected by tea, do not take tea when you are about to go to bed.

4. If your insomnia is because of the pains, get proper treatment for that pain.

5. And if worries have become your enemy, and causing you lack of sleep, try your best to solve those problems that are causing you worries. You must also know that by mere worries, you are not going to solve your problems. Whatever problem you might have, try to work hard on the solutions, and also engage other people to help you solve the problems, or else you are heading for serious health problems. Besides, know that everybody alive, has problems. There is absolutely no body alive without problems of any kind.

   And as you go to sleep, try your best to shut your mind to those problems. Also know that worrying at night while in your bed, is extremely dangerous. Because at that time of the night, you have nothing to do to occupy you, except to concentrate in your worries. And as you get deeply involved in your worries, your heart may be overpowered, and you get heart attack easily. And if it does not kill you, then it would have left you yet with another problem to worry about.

   So stop worrying, but work out the solutions, for there is no problem without a solution. Another thing is that, you may be worrying over something that may not even happen anyway, deception. Even though it may come about as per your fear, yet even this will pass away. Be at peace and let GOD handle those problems if you cannot handle them. Do not kill yourself, prematurely.

CHAPTER 16- TEMPER

Temper can be our own biggest enemy, if we do not control it. Hot temper has destroyed and killed a lot of people. And people who have uncontrolled hot temper are prone to heart attacks. Even if you do not have heart attack, you may still create for yourself some other health problems, such as severe headache, chest pains, high and rapid heartbeat which is not good for your heart, etc. Because of continuous hot temper, you may also end up with high blood pressure.

These emotional induced illness that you may develop, will in long run ground you down. You may become unable to do anything, totally disabled. And as you become disabled, means you will have to depend on other people for help. And your dependence on other people is not only a nuisance, but will also depress you much more, considering that you were once totally independent.

Let us now look into details, the problems hot temper may create for you.

PROBLEMS HOT TEMPER CAN CAUSE YOU

There are quite a lot of problems hot temper can cause you. And some of these are:

1. HEART ATTACK

Hot temper can cause you heart attack. And this may kill you instantly as has been the case with many people. If you survive the death by heart attack, your health may no longer be normal in most cases. And if however you happen to recover, you should be careful of subsequent heart attack because this may surely kill you.

STROKE

If you do not get heart attack from hot temper, you may get a stroke. This is equally worse, because it will paralyze you. Sometimes both your legs and your hands become totally paralyzed. You will not be able to work nor to lift your hands. And sometimes the whole body may become paralyzed. That means even sitting will become affected. You will not be able to sit. Turning your body while in bed may also become affected, and what that means, is that you will not be able to turn your body independently, you will need the help of other people to turn your body.

Your speech and memory may also become grossly affected. You may no longer be able to speak, and if you are able to, your speech may become fully distorted. And your memory may become totally impaired.

CAUSE YOU TO FIGHT

Hot temper may also cause you to fight as you may no longer tolerate the behaviour of other people or their arguments.

HOT TEMPER MAY CAUSE YOU TO KILL

Hot temper may also drive you to kill. When you flare into rage, you become totally intoxicated by that rage and unable to control yourself, hence you will do the things that you would not do under normal circumstances.

HOT TEMPER CAN SEND YOU TO PRISON

If you hurt or kill someone as a result of hot temper, you next destination, surely, will be the prison.

HOT TEMPER CAN MAKE YOU LOSE FRIENDS

Because of hot temper, you may lose your friends. As you flare into rage, you might say something bad to your friend that you normally do not say. You may even end up fighting them.

HOT TEMPER CAN DESTROY YOUR FAMILY

You may lose your family because of hot temper. As hot temper inhabits you and conquers you, you will fight with your family members on issues that do not warrant even an argument.

HOT TEMPER MAY CAUSE YOU TO HAVE AN ACCIDENT

Let say you are driving and there is a passenger in the car with you, and you happened to pick up an argument. You flew into rage and thereby immediately lost control of yourself as well of the car. On quite a busy road, you may end up knocking a crossing pedestrian, ram into another vehicle, a pole, a ditch, etc. as the argument heats up.

HOT TEMPER MAY CAUSE YOU TO BE HURT

Because of hot temper, you may be hurt by other people.

HOT TEMPER CAN CAUSE YOU DEATH

Hot temper may also cause you to be killed by other people.

HOT TEMPER MAY CAUSE YOU TO COMMIT OTHER CRIMES

When you are in rage, you may commit crimes you had never intended to commit.

HOT TEMPER MAY ALSO CAUSE YOU TO MISTREAT A WRONG POERSON

Because you became mad with someone, you might wrongfully take that rage onto someone totally innocent, e.g. an employee under you, a family member, a child, a friend, etc.

HOT TEMPOER MAY INTERFER WITH YOUR BLOOD CIRCULATION

Hot temper will interrupt your normal blood circulation.

HOT TEMPER WILL CAUSE YOU IMMEDIATE HEADACHE

Hot temper will cause you immediate severe headache.

CHEST PAIN

Hot temper can also cause you immediate chest pain.

HOT TEMPER CAN INTERRUPT THE NORMAL FUNCTION OF YOUR SEXUAL ORGAN

Hot temper can also interfere with your normal sexual functions. And if it is not put under control and occurs frequently for a continuous period, it may cause huge sexual problems.

HOT TEMPER CAN INTERFERE WITH YOUR BODY FUNCTION

Your body normal function can also be interfered with by hot temper. And if it continues for a long time, it may have severe consequences on your health. It may also lead to death.

SOLUTIONS

It is very difficult to get rid of hot temper, especially if it had been in you for a very long time. However try the following:

1. When you see that you are about to develop hot temper, simply walk away.

2. Stay away from the place of argument and the person at least for an hour. Return only when you have regained your cool.

3. Visualize the possible serious consequences. Think of the possible worst one.

4. Go talk to the friend you like.

5. In case you are driving and the argument was with a passenger, immediately find a parking spot and park the car there for a while. Move away from that passenger also for a while and return to the car only when you have cooled down and never begin any talk with that passenger.

CHAPTER 17- MORNING RELAXATION

When you get out of bed, early morning relaxation is critical for you. It is like laying a foundation of a house. If you lay a mediocre foundation, you know for sure that, that house is not going to last for long. It will collapse midway when you are not yet ready to move somewhere else, hence leaving you in unexpected problems.

It is the same with early morning relaxation. You do not want to start your day on a wrong note, do you? Therefore, when you wake up, leave the problems of yesterday into yesterday, and leave the problems of the night into the night, and begin a new chapter with a new day that The Lord has made.

Start right on a happy note with high expectation and The Lord's joy and happiness. Do not begin the morning with mourning, worries and unhappiness, otherwise you will ruin the whole day.

That day will bring you nothing but misery, pains, headaches, and much more problems that you worry over and not yet worry over. For you get what you expect.

When you are from your bed, feel good and energized. Proclaim the great new day and begin to be glad and happy in it. Make yourself happy and know and believe that GOD ALMIGHTY is in full control of everything and every situation, here on earth and in heaven. Wish for the best in your life that day. Proclaim great things for that day. And remove sadness from your face for it is a new day.

Also know that life is a complete mystery, and we do not have control over it, what is to happen will happen. We cannot stop anything from happening and whatever is destined for us. So be happy, come rain, come sun shine. And remember good things attract good things and bad things attract bad things, and bad thoughts attract bad things.

CHAPTER 18- SMELL

The body reacts differently to different kinds of smell. It may like some smell and at the same time it may hate others. In other words, the body gets affected by different smell. Sometimes the body immediately resists certain smell by sneezing. And some other smell may cause us chest pain and sometimes difficulty in breathing.

Smell in general can be good and at the same time be terribly bad. Smell of certain foods for example may instantly arouse our appetite, while others may immediately send us sick. And this can even be worse if we are allergic to this kind of smell. It may kill us instantly.

There are however, different kinds of smell. The smell of foods that we have already seen above, and the smell of other things.

KINDS OF SMELL AND THEIR EFFECTS

As stated above, there are different kinds of smell. And these are:

1. SMELL OF FOODS

   We have already partially talked about this above. Anyhow, let look at some of these into details.

   Certain people are allergic to some kinds of food smell. It does not only disturb them, but also cause them to become sick or even instantly die.

2. CHEMICAL SMELL

   Chemical smell is poisonous. If you inhale this for long, you will not only become sick, but will die.

   SEWAGE SMELL

   Sewage smell can be very annoying and toxic at the same time. Prolonged smell of this may cause us to become sick.

   GARBAGE SMELL

   Garbage smell can also be toxic due to the fermentation of different stuffs. Its smell is not only irritating but can also become a source of health problems.

VEHICLE SMOKE SMELL

This is very toxic and we should be very careful with it and should never expose ourselves to it for too long.

ORDINARY SMOKE SMELL

This is also a health hazard as it may cause health problems if inhaled for long.

THEIR EFFECTS

a. Some of this smell may cause us to become sick.

b. We may develop respiratory problems.

c. May in the long run affect our lungs and weakens their normal functions.

d. May affect our kidneys.

e. May cause death.

PREVENTION

1. When you are always exposed to smell of dangerous chemicals, remember always to wear a mask.

2. Move away from that area that is contaminated by the smell.

3. If inhaled, seek immediate medical attention.

4. If the smell is in the house, open all the windows and leave the house immediately.

CHAPTER 19- GOD ALMIGHTY

Above all, there is GOD ALMIGHTY who has absolute authority over everything, living and none-living, dead and alive, seen and unseen. HE also has full authority over your health, life and your life-span. And HE decides everything about you.

GODS AUTHORITY

You can be eating well, exercising everyday, taking care of yourself, but if GOD decides that you will not be well, then definitely you will not be well. And if HE decides that despite the good health you have, you will suddenly die, nothing, will stop that from happening.

This does not mean GOD is cruel as other people normally tend to think. No, GOD is never cruel otherwise we should all have been dead because of the many sins in our lives. GOD is good and merciful all the times.

GOD is the knowledge itself. HE is yesterday, today and tomorrow. HE is eternal with absolute powers. He sees everything that comes your way. Besides, HE is never wrong. If GOD ALMIGHTY decides that you die today, it is not cruelty, because HE may be saving you from the worst horrible things coming your way. Instead of leaving you to terribly suffer, HE says, my child come over. But for us, human beings, we look at it the wrong way. Remember, GOD is never wrong and HE does not undertake the trial and err process, for HE knows and is always precise in all HIS decisions and undertakings.

SEEK HIM FIRST

Always seek HIM, honour HIM, adore HIM and pray to HIM that it will always be well with you.

If you honour GOD ALMIGHTY, all will be well with you. Sickness will flee from you, poverty will flee from you, sufferings will flee from you, and the list is totally endless. However, the problem with the human beings, is that we tend to honour ourselves, and acknowledge that we exist and GOD does not. What ignorance! We also think that we are the masters over our problems and destinies, yet most of the times, we cannot solve even the most minute problems, in our lives. And if we are not able to solve even the smallest problems, then how are we able to solve big and complicated one!

Always take your problems to him who has the clues to all problems. Problems to HIM are not problems, small or big, regardless.

Regarding life and health, some of the guidelines are in HIS words. The problems of health and life are most of the times, our own creation as a result of disobedience of HIS TEN COMMANDMENTS. And yet there is life and protection in them. When we disobey them, we are virtually putting curses into our lives. And curses can range from sickness to death, from lack to abject poverty, from worries to depression, or complete madness.

The word of GOD is also clear about life and sins. It clearly states that the reward of sins is death. And if we sin, then we are getting closer to death. It is the physical death and never the spiritual death as you hear some preachers say, for the spirit does not die and it is the physical body that dies. That is why there is hell to punish the living wicked spirits.

This notion is crystal clear, if you are caught stealing and you are killed, it is the body that is killed and not the spirit. And if you are caught committing adultery and you are killed, it is the body that is killed and not the spirit. That wicked spirit that led you to steal or commit adultery remains alive and his thrown into GOD's prison, hell, to be punished. It remains alive forever but under punishments.

So as you can see, the word of GOD is right, when we sin we invite death into our lives. We also invite sickness into our lives. We invite sickness into our lives, for example if we go about fornicating, and we happen to meet a wrong person, he or she may infect us with sexual diseases.

So to stay healthy and have a longevity, avoid sinning, for sins are the enemies of GOD.

PROTECTION, GOOD HEALTH, BLESSINGS AND LONGEVITY

PROTECTION

For your own protection from those things, seen and unseen, you need GODs protection always. Because you on your own can not provide yourself full protection.

GOOD HEALTH

We may eat well, drink well, exercise from January 01 to December 31, and yet if GOD is not with us, it is vanity. We can become sick or even die. It is GOD ALMIGHTY who gives us good health. And if you are eating well, drinking well, exercising well, etc. it is still HIM making you get all those good foods, drinks, and good health to exercise. All these things are HIS own making and never yours.

BLESSINGS

The blessings that GOD ALMIGHTY bestows into your life, will afford you happiness, and happiness will translate into good health and longevity.

LONGEVITY

Who has authority over longevity, you, us human beings? Longevity comes from GOD ALMIGHTY HIMSELF. HE decides how long you are going to live. If GOD decides that you live up to two hundred years or more, who can stop that from happening. It will happen regardless. And in all those years if HE wants you to remain healthy to the end, you will, regardless. GOD is absolute authority.

DO NOT DO BAD THINGS TO OTHERS

To avoid curses and bad things that may happen to you, avoid altogether doing bad things to other people. Remember, everybody is created by GOD HIMSELF, we all belong to HIM, black or white, blue or green, pink or purple, we are all HIS, so be careful or you may set yourself against GOD.

If you do bad things to other people, they cry to GOD and GOD listens to their cries and takes revenge. And when GOD tames you, you will think twice before you again hurt other people.

www.ingramcontent.com/pod-product-compliance
Lightning Source LLC
Chambersburg PA
CBHW020336290526
45785CB00005B/2044